THE POWER OF

INTERMITTENT FASTING

Effortless diet for achieving long-term low body fat & mental toughness and building lean muscle (for men & women)

Written by

Matej Kacvisnky

Author of : „Naturally boost your testosterone" and „Yoga for men"

„Be able to fully enjoy your diet so it becomes so easy there is no willpower, because that´s how you are going to win in the long run."

„The most common mistake why people do not achieve low body fat is the lack of consistency."

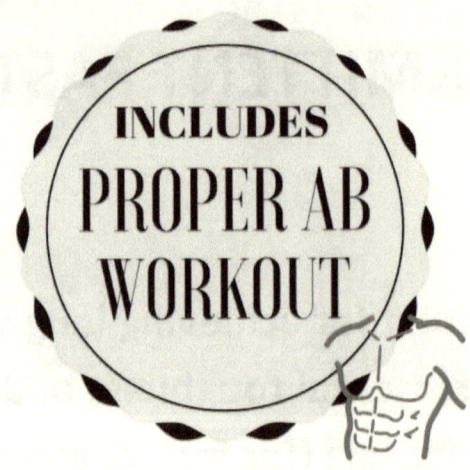

Contents

Introduction

Do you want to get really lean without having to kill yourself every time you deny yourself the foods that you enjoy the most? Do you want to make your diet effortless as possible? In this book I will gladly offer you solutions on how to stop this mental battle that is just brutal and make your dieting enjoyable and rewarding. That's what life should be about right? I see so many people struggle with fasting and that's the last thing that fasting should be about.

The book subheading clearly accentuates the word effortless. But how to get to this point of effortless dieting? First, let me tell you this: We are always told to eat every 3 hours to keep our metabolism and protein synthesis running and the reality is that research doesn't prove that in the slightest. It doesn't matter if you have one meal or 10 meals. Your metabolism is dictated by many different factors and eating itself is just one factor and it has no bearing over how often you eat. It's a matter of how much you eat, so when you eat 2000 calories in a day, your body is going to burn the same amount of calories whether it was in one meal or ten meals.

The reality is, when you do intermittent fasting - stop

eating breakfast and push your first meal later into the day, your growth hormone goes through the roof. The research shows, there is a 2000% increase of growth hormone in men and 1200% in women. That growth hormone actually helps shuttle fat cells into the blood stream, which will be burned for energy.

We have to think about this for a second. With the same genetic code as a hunter-gatherer ancestors we thrived on very little food in the morning. We had to go hunt in the morning so our body is well designed to be very efficient in a fasted state. It triggers the sympathetic nervous system, which makes you focused, alert and energetic. Contrarily if you have a huge meal like an oatmeal, and fruits or bread early in the morning your blood sugar gets a huge spike and what happens...? You feel sluggish, tired and hungry 2 hours later. That's why we are programmed to eat very little during the day, fast and really maximize the fat burning, which will keep you in that laser-focused state and to feast at night like our ancestors did around a big fireplace.

Your doctor might say to you, that it is not the healthiest way how to eat from today health perspective, where you are required to eat every couple hours, because you don't want to devote yourself to any kind of eating disorder right? However he can't tell you this thing – that it is not going to be efficient for building an amazing body, lean muscle and burning your fat effortlessly.

It is known, that eating disorders are mainly a matter of psychological issues and are strongly connected with experiencing shame, guilt and low self-esteem as an individual. It's a sad truth...

If you are now thinking, that you can evocate eating disorder because of intermittent fasting you are just getting a little bit paranoid.

In addition to that, there is also no proof of getting an eating disorder from doing intermittent fasting 3-4 times a week for couple weeks or even months. It is mainly individual and it depends on your body adaptation ability as well. One person can gain great results from it while it doesn't really serve the other person.

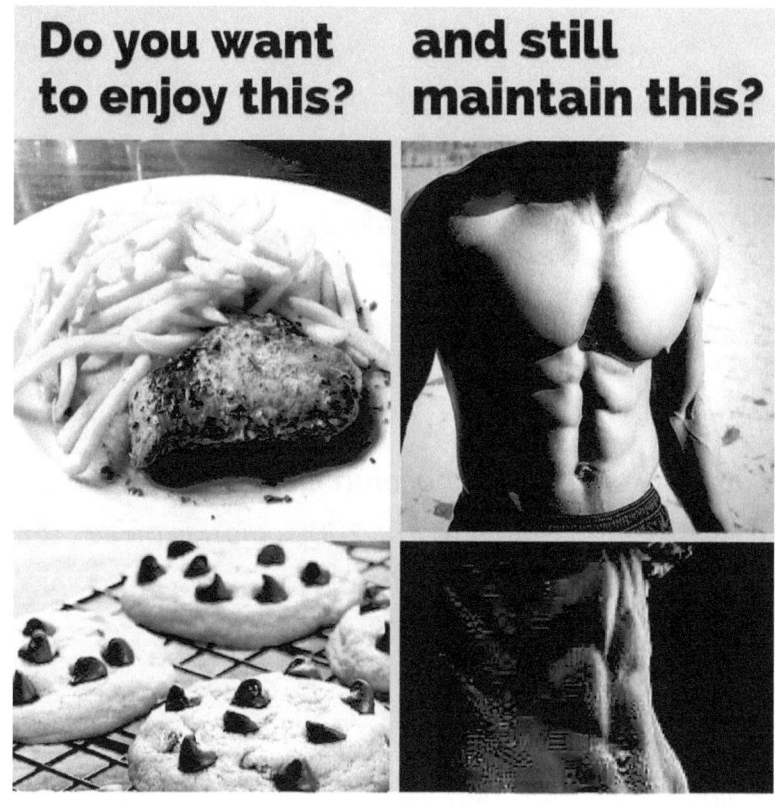

From my personal experience and experience of many of my clients I can say, that if a diet is not rewarding and is boring, you are going to make your life a hell of a lot harder, because you are going to get cravings. To be honest, you and I are only humans and we are going to cheat eventually, when a diet drains our willpower out. After that we usually feel guilty and that will make us overeat even more.

But you know what? If you are smart about this, you

can actually enjoy your chocolate or ice cream on a diet!
Sure, you won´t be able to eat 1000 calories of ice cream
or chocolate, but you can still enjoy it, while being in
a daily calorie deficit!

If you do like this idea, then you should read further,
because it is possible! I simply want as many people as
possible to know about this!

Chapter 1: Benefits and side effects of fasting

Fasting allows your body to rest. In fact the father of natural medicine – Hippocrates practiced fasting himself and back then it counted as the number one treatment for his patients. If you read the Bible, you´ll find out that fasting had been used as a way to spiritual enlightenment and health benefits for years as well. Nowadays lots of doctors and studies confirm, that intermittent fasting can naturally boost our hormones, weight loss, let our gut rest, support detoxification and healing.

If you struggle with things like constipation or diarrhea or any sort of bowel issues like leaky gut syndrome, intermittent fasting can definitely be beneficial.

Better vision while fasting?

Yes. But I discovered it accidentally. I have been wearing my contact lenses for about 6-7 years now. It was during one winter, when I noticed that my vision was not so sharp and accurate as it used to be.
I blamed lack of vitamin D and sun at first, because it is proven that vitamin D can make an impact on your vision (besides vitamin A which is more well-known). After not eating in the morning and going straight to work I experienced some noticeable improvements in my vision. I told everybody I knew, who wore glasses or used contact lenses back then and believe me or not 70% claimed sharper vision and being able to see brighter and crisper! People, who have naturally healthy eyesight won't notice as much of a change. There isn't much science behind it yet, because it doesn't seem to completely recover your eyesight and the boost in vision seems to be also just temporary.

Side effects and warning

Everything has to be done in moderation and it is especially true when it comes down to intermittent fasting. It is suggested to try it out for about 30-90 days to get major health benefits. Fasting is created for being done on a periodic basis, not for an entire life. It is a perfect tool for leaning down before summer, competition, as a heart disease prevention or just toughening up. Use it, get the benefits and come back to it again in the future.

First couple of days of doing intermittent fasting can make you feel anxious, angry or even little bit tired but don't worry, it won't take any longer than 2-3 days. Your mood can be low during those days, however it is not always like that. There is a proof, that your mood becomes even more positive than before, after your body has adapted to the fasted state. It is not recommended for pregnant women and people with diabetes though.

Chapter 2: Spiritual side of dieting

Are you one of those people, who transforms himself into a cortisol-producing stress machine when it comes to dieting? Alright, don´t worry, because you are not alone. I see so many people making this mistake over and over, which totally sabotages all of their chances to persist further in their diet. I used to be like that too.

Stressing out about your diet won´t do any good to you, but rob you of all your willpower. You will feel down and without energy to do other things like taking care of your daily job, kids, buying groceries, having a great time meeting your friends, surprising your husband, wife or spouse and doing something for yourself.

Let me introduce you my diet ideology. It is not „mine" indeed, but I got inspired by one of the modern spiritual teachers – Eckhart Tolle. He claims, that life should be experienced and enjoyed in this very moment.

Do you agree so far? People always ask me things like: „What are you biggest regrets in life?" and I say to them „I don´t know." – I simply don´t think about that, because it just doesn´t make sense to take something that isn´t and let it affect something that is. I know – these are kind of spiritual thought processes, but do you get the idea? The point of that is, that when you are eating, you are eating and when you are fasting, you are fasting and you enjoy both activities the same.

How can I enjoy both the same, are you serious? Yes. Both of them bring different advantages. If you are eating, you enjoy the food that is melting on your tongue and deriving the pleasure out of it. However if you are fasting, you can experience a state of alertness and focus, which will allow you to get things done and be productive during your day. This will also give you a feeling of enjoyment and satisfaction and make you feel great about yourself at the end of the day. It will make your work matter and you will appreciate what you have done. Being on intermittent fasting further correlates with feelings of increased self-importance and self-esteem. Don´t believe me? Try it for yourself.

Chapter 3: The main idea of fasting

There are many types of fasting methods like 16/8 and 20/4 method or Eat/Stop/Eat method. For example 16/8 means that you go 16 hours without eating (sleep included) and you eat for about +/- 8 hours. „What´s the best method for me to use?"– You might ask. The one that is the easiest for you to keep consistently. That is especially important in the beginning, when your body is not used to it yet. So which one? Don´t take it so dogmatically. Let me put it this way...

First of all push your first meal later into the day so you can get that increasing growth hormone and increasing fat burning. First days try to do it as long as you can – maybe even 2-3 hours for the start, but your goal are at least 6 hours after you wake up until your first meal. All the bodybuilders and fitness enthusiasts, who want to build muscle mass and are afraid of catabolism I want to tell, that the growth hormone released while you are fasting actually protects your muscle mass so you are not going to be burning your muscle. You are going to tap right into the fat storage because growth hormone is needed and required to accelerate the fat burning. That's why is a great way for lean bulking!

For now, please forget about the eating window during the day you are used to. I recommend – again - to eat around 6 hours after you wake up. Imagine yourself not eating a single calorie 6 or even 8 hours after you become awake. After you have been fasting for about – let's say those 6 hours, you have about 8 hours to eat foods that you enjoy. Well, think about how enjoyable dieting is going to be for you, because now you get this small 8 hour window, when you can eat a lot of food. However those 8 hours can be more or less depending on your preference and circumstances. For instance: You have had your first meal at 1 pm and you came home later at 10 or 11 pm and you are below your calorie deficit (I will show you how to calculate your deficit in Chapter 10), feel free to enjoy your food before you go to bed.

You might ask - Is eating before falling asleep going to be healthy? I am going to talk about it in a moment but first let me comment on some practical side of intermittent fasting.

Chapter 4: Practicality of fasting

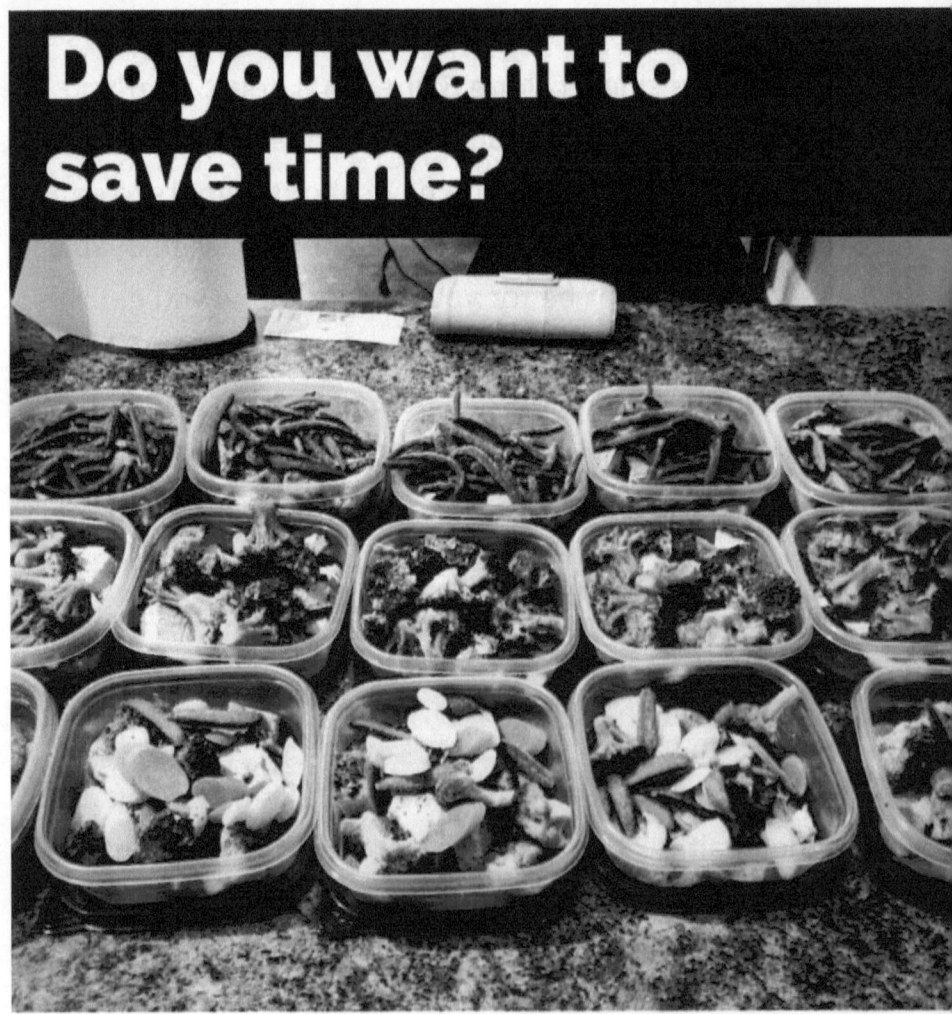

Imagine yourself going several hours into the day without even thinking about food or having to prepare any meal. Preparing or cooking food has to perfectly suit your daily schedule. You should feel relaxed and enjoy doing it. You shouldn't be cooking your food like a robot every 3-4 hours just to keep your mind from getting paranoid and feeling guilty that you are not getting enough proteins every 3 hours.

I don't recommend to have an exact starting time when you eat your first meal after your fasting period. That's just too strict. You don't need that. Why should you have so many rules around your eating? Listen to your body but most importantly try to push those first 6 hours without eating every day for maximal results (it's an important rule – that's why I keep repeating it over and over). At the end of the day it is about hitting those calories. I have to laugh when I see people or cookbooks offering you 100+ recipes for intermittent fasting. May I ask, what for? It is like offering you 100 recipes for eating what you want.

Intermittent fasting is not about restricting what you eat but when and how much of it you eat. So you don't need any special recipes – hell, you don't even have to cook! Here are some delicious food examples you can snack on without having to cook them when doing intermittent fasting:

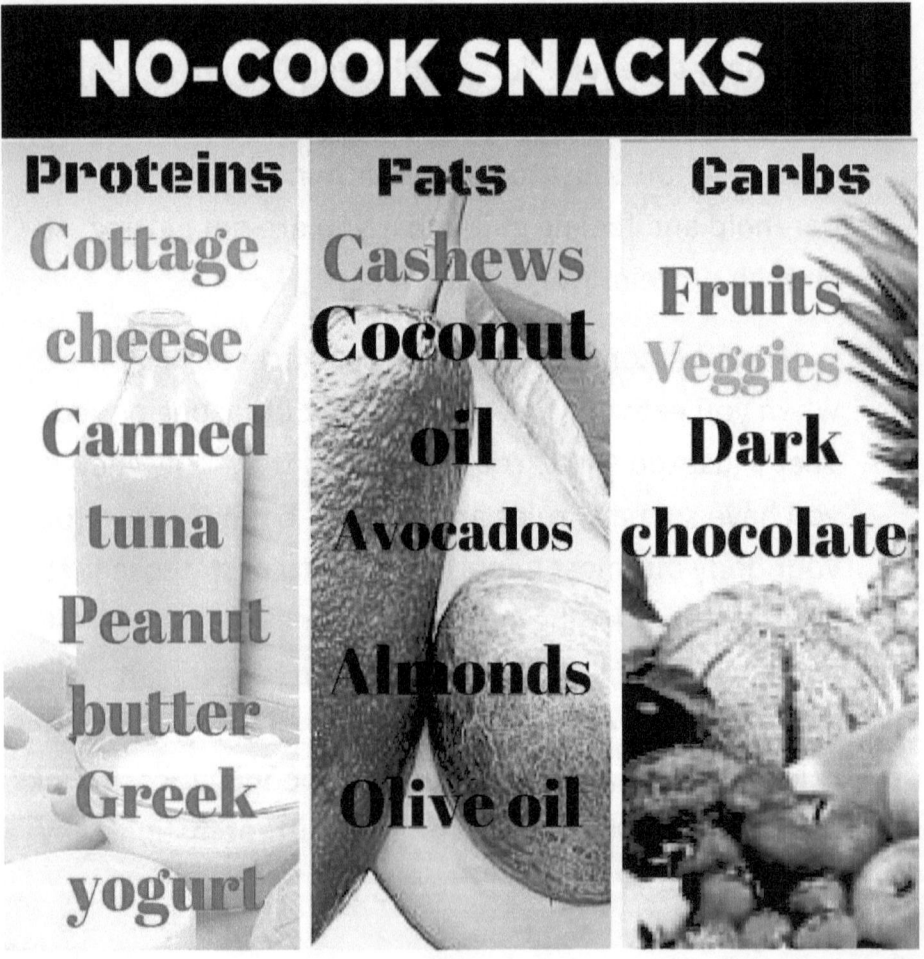

The only thing you need is to enjoy what you like to

eat, however do it strategically.

Isn´t it weird and unhealthy going without eating for such a long time?

Not necessarily. Your body is actually designed to function well in a fasted state. Your body is going to kick up energy through increasing fat burning so you´ll have all the energy you need while doing fasting. It´s going to be more than enough energy to „survive" your first half of the day in your job or anywhere else – trust me.

Forget about that you are fasting. It´s not a big deal. The more you think about it the harder it is going to be for you. Trust me, it is highly rewarding as long as you let it be rewarding and not trying to think way to much about it.

Chapter 5: Fasting and caffeine

As intermittent fasting itself, caffeine has to be used strategically as well. There are many people who don´t drink coffee or drink simply too much of it. You want to strike the balance. If you try to fast without any additional caffeine, you are making it a lot harder on yourself. Coffee will actually amplify the fasting because it spreads those stored fat cells into the blood stream. This way you will burn your fat for energy. This process increases the norepinephrine synthesis which causes your arousal and alertness to increase, promotes vigilance, enhances formation and retrieval of memory, and focuses attention.

One issue that I see is that people drink too much coffee. If you drink coffee many times during the day, guess what - you are not going to be sensitive to caffeine and it is going to be suppressing your appetite. You want to be drinking your coffee during the fast only and no other time. That will keep your body sensitive to the caffeine and blunt your appetite effectively while fasting, which will in the end make fasting very easy.

If you don´t like coffee you can choose green tea as well. I love to drink it for many other reasons than its caffeine presence. It has been proven, that green tea helps you with fat loss especially around your stomach and keeps your teeth whiter unlike coffee. Green tea or coffee? I think, there are more milligrams of caffeine in a coffee that in a green tea, I experienced similar results from both though. I´ll leave it up to you.

Chapter 6: Drinking enough water

This is one very powerful trick that will help you make your fasting really effortless and you won´t be even thinking about food. Simply drink more water, which will promote detoxification and cleansing when drinking on empty stomach. It can be soda or carbonated water as well. That will fill up your empty stomach in the morning. There are also lots of benefits of drinking sparkling water like high mineral profile.

When you are fasting for a while and only drinking water, your liver glycogen will become depleted and that will send a signal to your brain to "make you hungry." You can actually shut that signal off by replenishing a little bit of your liver glycogen and the way you do that is with fruit, because fruit is made up of fructose and glucose and the fructose helps replenish the liver glycogen. So having something like an apple or banana at the end of your fast when you start to get hungry, can be really effective at staving off hunger.

More importantly, fruit is actually best consumed on an empty stomach from my experience, because you want to eat fruit when carbohydrate stores are low. If you've had a big meal and you eat a piece of fruit on the top of that, your liver glycogen stores will be topped off so that fruit will either have to be burned for energy or stored as fat. And I don't know many people who like to have cardio right after eating a big meal so guess what – Calories from fruits consumed on a full stomach will eventually be converted into fat.

The second reason, why to consume fruits on an empty stomach is, that it will be absorbed better. For example, if you wake up at 7 am, you may grab some piece of fruit at around 12 am or 1 pm. That way you will be sated for another hour or two before you'll eat your first meal.

Chapter 7: Strategies on having your 1st and last meal after your fasting period

Your first meal should be the greatest reward of the day and fully satiate you. Don´t force yourself to do something that doesn´t feel right. After not eating for the first 6-8 hours of the day, the most unnatural thing would be restricting yourself in your first meal. Usually I literally eat foods I like as a part of my first meal – potatoes, french-fries, lean meat, dark chocolate, burger and some veggies. You can eat those foods high in calories, because you simply have the room to work with. I try to have a prevalent part of my proteins contained in my first meal – that way I won´t get "paranoid" about things like having enough proteins during my day. However, if you are afraid of losing muscle during sleep you can consume one Greek yogurt or cottage cheese in the evening/before sleep.

Eating late and before going to bed

After you had your first meal, you can have couple of snacks and then your second meal. I usually snack on some chocolate bar, cheesecake or some random things. Yes, I like to snack. However do, what feels right for you. You can even split it in 3 meals but I found out that it was rather time consuming.

Sometimes I eat right before going to bed – It´s completely fine. Some people say that eating before going to bed may cause insulin and growth hormone to release. However growth hormone will still be released anyways throughout the entire night, because it is released in a pulse-like fashion. It means, that if your insulin is high by falling asleep (usually because of eating a prevalent amount carbs), insulin will taper off eventually as you get the boost in growth hormone so there is really nothing to worry about. This will actually boost your muscle-building during the night.

Separating your carbs from your 1st meal

This tip is really worth a lot of money, because it helped me so much!

Let's say I am having a big 1st meal and I'll have something like a big stake with butter, cheese and veggies – pretty much everything but the carbs. That way I save my carbs for after. This will help me feel satiated longer. If I would give you a stake and fries, you might want to feel like eating some dessert or snacking on something after that. However if I'd give you just a stake, cheese and veggies and couple hours later some fries or rice, you wouldn't even need them as much anymore. Try it out – It works wonders!

Chapter 8: Intermittent fasting and cardio

You don't want to make fasting any harder than it is. If you are waking up in the morning and doing some intense workout like cross-fit or high intensity interval training as a first thing of the day —well, you are going to give yourself a ravenous appetite straight away and you are going to make fasting 10 times more difficult than it is. Focus your morning training on ab workout or aerobic if you like and do not burn yourself out faster and make yourself hungry.

Even additional 20 minutes of cardio is a lot when fasting! However it is a different thing if you do it at the end of the fast, because you will eat soon anyways.

Be careful with cardio, if you don't want to be starving from hunger soon. Now I only walk usually 30 to

60 minutes a day, which has made no impact on my appetite. That way you'll increase your bare calorie deficit in 200-300 calories without increasing your appetite. It means, that it will enable you to consume 200-300 more as you are allowed to. Hmm, maybe some delicious protein bar?

People usually think of cardio and exercising one-dimensionally. They just think about burning a specific amount of calories, but they don't look at the bigger picture...You have to ask, how does cardio affect my total daily calorie consumption? Cardio is actually pretty much useless and most unpractical thing, when it comes to intermittent fasting. It is just not efficient, because it will be counterproductive and can pretty much sabotage your willpower.

Let me put it this way – Maybe you are brave and start your day with cardio, because you think it's a healthy start of the day. Yes it sure is, but unless you haven't been doing cardio for months now so it could've become automatized you will have to use some willpower on pushing yourself to do it at first right? That exact willpower you used on your early cardio , you may miss later when you are thinking about eating some extra dessert. If you did too much cardio earlier, you won't have enough willpower to stop those cravings and you snack onto that dessert and you'll overeat.

However if you are an athlete, gymnast, swimmer, player of any kind of sports or you simply love cardio you can´t totally avoid it. Please remember that I am not saying – Don´t do cardio! Not at all. I represent a way of doing things smart not hard. That´s why just do not recommend doing cardio so you can spare yourself great amounts of time while still being able to lean down effectively without it.

Chapter 9: Intermittent fasting and working out

In the beginning I used to eat my first meal 1-2 hours before I hit the gym. I had been focused on eating enough, so it could've given me an amazing energy boost for working out but not too much that I would've felt stuffed in the gym.

Try to save the majority of your carbs after your workout. That way your body will use most of those carbs for anabolic processes like muscle and hormone-building processes rather than for pure fat storing.

When I do not eat for a whole day and I worked out, I do not experience weakness associated with fasting in my lifts. I feel the same as if I would have eaten. Don't worry you won't lose any muscle. As soon as you reach your calorie maintenance level for the day you will lose fat and keep your muscle.

Yes, it is true that if you work out in a fasted state for the first time you may feel like sh.t, because you are not used to it yet but the next time it will feel much better!

I am that kind of person, who likes to have something in his stomach before working out, however I´ve found out, that when I was training in a fasted state once, my energy levels and strength were even better. First time I was pretty discouraged to do it, but it felt incredible! Now, when I usually train, I train in fasted state. I can see an incredible increase of energy and alertness in the gym every time. This time, I usually film various videos and do some shots for youtube.com, because my muscle definition is better, I feel leaner and have much higher pleasure on working out. How can it be possible? Well, let me explain it. First, your body is in a catabolic state which enables fat burning. Second, it causes your energy hormones like adrenaline and cortisol to rise.

Another benefit of working out in a fasted state is, that you will drain your blood sugar. This will make you more insulin sensitive and which is really good! What does it mean? It simply means that when you do eat carbs straight after your training, they go straight into your muscle tissue and your muscle cells will use them for anabolic processes. Remember that by many people, who are not insulin sensitive and eat much carbs, those carbs will be stored as fat really quickly.

You want to eat big, otherwise your meals won't provide enough nutrients that you need. I am giving you permission to eat a lot more than seems reasonable after your training. As long as you count your calories and macros (I will show you how to do that exactly in the 11th Chapter) and know how much you have to reach, everything is going to be fine.

I know so many people who are afraid of eating big especially during the evening time thinking they are going to gain fat from it. However, as long as you are aware of your calorie maintenance level and your macros are being taken care of it really doesn't matter. If you are in that deficit, you will drop that fat for sure! Just because you are eating such a big portion of the meal and you might even feel little stuffed after that you are not going to be storing fat. That's not how fat loss works. It's about the numbers. Keep that in mind.

Chpater 10: How does fat loss work?

As far as building a great physique, it is a matter of building a proper muscle development and a matter of getting really lean. When you have very little fat on your body, that´s when you have a great definition. Even your face is chiseled and angular, your muscles have more separation, because there is no fat which could „stay in the way." That´s the point, when your muscles start to pop out. As I noted before, great muscle definition can be amplified while working out in a fasted state. That´s why many bodybuilders do not eat and only drink water before posing on stage.

Having low body fat consistently is a matter of achieving calorie deficit, so when you eat less calories than your body burns, that's what causes you to get rid of the fat around your body. You can simply frame the previous sentence and put it above your bed, because it is really the cardinal rule to fat loss. That said, you can eat the foods that you enjoy as long as you stick to the numbers. Fat loss is a numbers game, it's about getting an optimal amount of protein, fats and carbs but you can include your favorite foods in it.

Chapter 11: Macronutrients and calorie calculator

You don't need to track your macros if you want to lean down. You don't have to obsessively count how much fat, carbs and protein you eat every single meal. I can tell you that it is much easier if you let go of tracking everything. However the most important thing is having a sufficient amount of protein and I want to tell you in a moment, what that ideal amount is.

If you spend all your mental energy on trying to make everything perfectly fit to your macros you simply deplete your willpower reserves on pointless things, you could have used on things like doing an additional work for your job, writing a blog post or an article, spend more quality time with your friends or family or as simple as reading some good book.

You can comfortably forget about all those macronutrient ratios like 50-30-20 or 40-40-20 (stands for percentages of protein, carbohydrates and fat). It's just too much noise you don´t need. You want to consume around 0,8 grams of protein per pound of bodyweight or 1,8 g per kg of bodyweight. That´s literally all you need! After that make sure that you eat anything you enjoy with high nutritional value until you reach your daily calorie deficit.

After I make sure my protein macros are being taken care of for the day, I aim next for more of those healthy fats like avocado, cashews, olive oil, coconut oil, even bacon with plenty of butter, cheese and some carbs, which I get from potato chips, fries and fruits, dark chocolate and some cookies. You don´t want to forget about balanced carb-fat ratio, because it helps us balance our hormones and increase testosterone. However I do not count my carbohydrate and fat macros. I simply focus that I consume a sufficient amount of calories to achieve my daily calorie deficit. It makes my life a lot easier and I hope that it will make yours as well!

How to find out my calorie deficit?

Glad you ask. To make it easier for you, I am just going to give you some links for calculating your calorie maintenance level. I personally use calculator.net most of the time, but you can find many other calculators on the internet.

*CML – calorie maintenance level

Click here to see your current CML
http://www.calculator.net/calorie-calculator.html

Calorie calculator is really amazing! First, you have to complete your gender, age, weight and height information. Important field is your activity level, because this is going to have an impact on your overall calorie deficit. If two persons of the same weight, height, gender and age have different activity levels – let's say sedentary vs extra active, you can be sure that there is going to be an additional buffer of 1500 calories, which the second person can eat to reach his maintenance level in comparison to the first person with a sedentary way of life.

The more often you work out, the higher your calorie deficit will be. After you hit calculate, it will show you what your current calorie maintenance level is and how much calories you can/have to eat for gaining/losing 1-2 pounds a week (1 pound = 0,45 kg). That's it guys! It's as easy as that.

However it can happen, that you are not losing/gaining as much weight on a weekly basis as you would like to. This happens to me sometimes as well. Here I would simply adjust my daily calorie deficit level in about +/- 100-200 calories and see what will happen in the next week. It is not an exact science and you have to play with it a little bit and watch how your body reacts to such calorie changes.

Chapter 12: Abdominals

Have you ever seen a person around 20% of body fat with defined abdominals? You are right – me neither. Imagine your abs like your facial muscles. There are around 42 muscles on your face. If you lose some fat in general, you will notice your face getting a nicer shape (if you are a man, your chin tends to look more edgy and masculine).

It simply doesn't matter how much you chew, smile or use your facial muscles, you won't burn fat on your face with it, because in the end it comes down to your overall body fat. It is exactly the same with your whole body. It can be chest, abs, legs or shoulders – doesn't matter. Do you get it?

Remember, that the only reason to work out your abs is to get stronger abs and that's what you will get too! It won't help you get rid of your belly fat. If you are interested in strengthening your abs, I recommend that you read all the commandments below. However if you just want to lose your belly fat, you can skip this section without any regrets and make losing your overall body fat your main priority instead.

Ab commandments

1. Get rid of fat in general

You can not get rid of your abdominal fat by doing ab exercises. This absurd saying would imply that working out your biceps will make you get rid of your fat around the biceps, which isn't true at all. It will only increase your strength or endurance of your muscle tissue in that particular area.

2. Work out your abs like other body parts

Abs are no different, than your triceps, chest or shoulders and you shouldn't be working them out more than 2-3 times a week. Do you know the theory of marginal returns? It works wonders, when it comes to exercising your abs or any other body part as well. It means, that with every additional ab workout you will get less and less additional results. Remember that your abs are being used almost all the time when you do squats, deadlifts, pull-ups or even push-ups. Instead of doing some additional sets of ab workout you find on the internet, use your willpower rather on fasting properly and keeping your calories under control.

3. **Focus on great form, lower repetitions and maximizing strength.**

Do you usually squat 4 sets of 100 repetitions or bench 4 sets of 30 repetitions? No. If you have to do 100 sit ups to feel your abdominals pumped, it just means that you are not working them out properly. You want to have strong abdominals, which will support your back by squatting and deadlifting and help you increase your core strength. I had made that mistake years ago before I have started with fitness. The results were none. I was doing countless repetitions with a sloppy form without any concentration on my abdominals. It was more like cardio, because back then I was doing my crunches so fast. It was a result of zero willpower to actually do them and I just wanted it all to be over soon.

Having strong abs is a foundation for movement throughout your entire body and foundation for injury prevention. It is important to perform slow movements for the muscles to contract properly. It is like squats – If you you have something around 140 kg or 300 pounds on your back and you have to squat it, you won´t probably move up that fast with your whole body – you will take your time, maybe even 4 seconds to bring yourself up.

You have to prepare your abs for such a long and continuous time under tension by exercising them properly.

Remember, if you work out your abs slowly and controlled, you let more muscle fibers be recruited to make the particular movement.
I recommend you to do 3 various ab exercises per session while doing 3 sets of 10-15 reps each. Do them properly and it´ll be more than you even need!

Chapter 13: BONUS: Abs Workout Routine – More is Less!

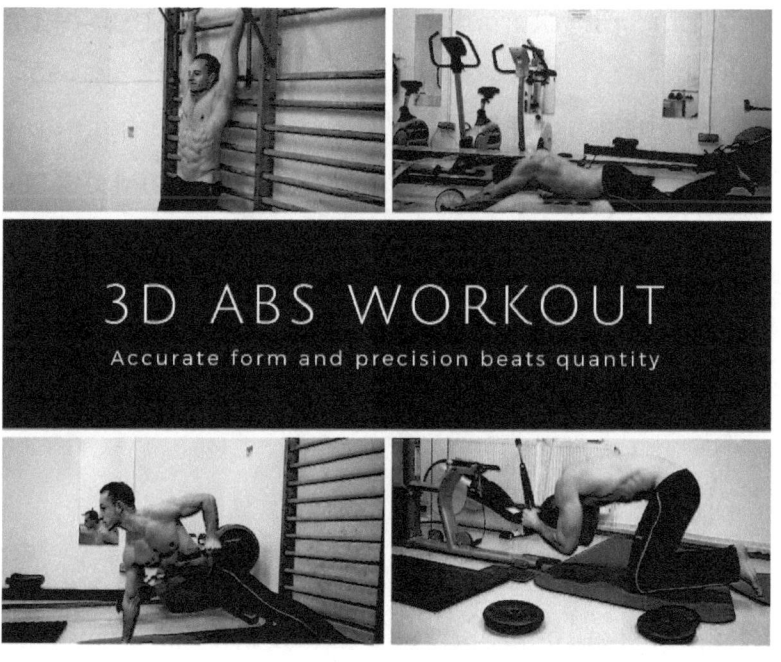

I have been practicing this work out routine for about 2 years with great success. I include the following abs routine in my trainings usually 3 times a week. I like to choose always 3 various exercises per workout and really focus on them. Again, it is not about how much you train but how precise you train it.   If you practice only 3 various ab exercises per training session, it can take you around 10-15 minutes to complete this workout while keeping proper form.

I still have a strong opinion that if you are around 15% - 20% body fat, you don´t have to work out your abs for burning your belly fat. It is simply a waste of time! On the other side, if you are around 7% - 12% you can make your abs look a hell of a lot better with proper ab training. I like to vary my ab routines from time to time and add some more advanced exercises to give my ab muscles new stimulation. Sometimes I like to practice human flag or planche push-ups which engages my abs in a totally different way.

Now forget about human flag and other advanced ab training routines and let´s take a brief look on the following exercises. I´d like to comment on some important things while we are going through them. I do 3 sets and 10-15 reps of each exercise and rest 30 seconds in between sets.

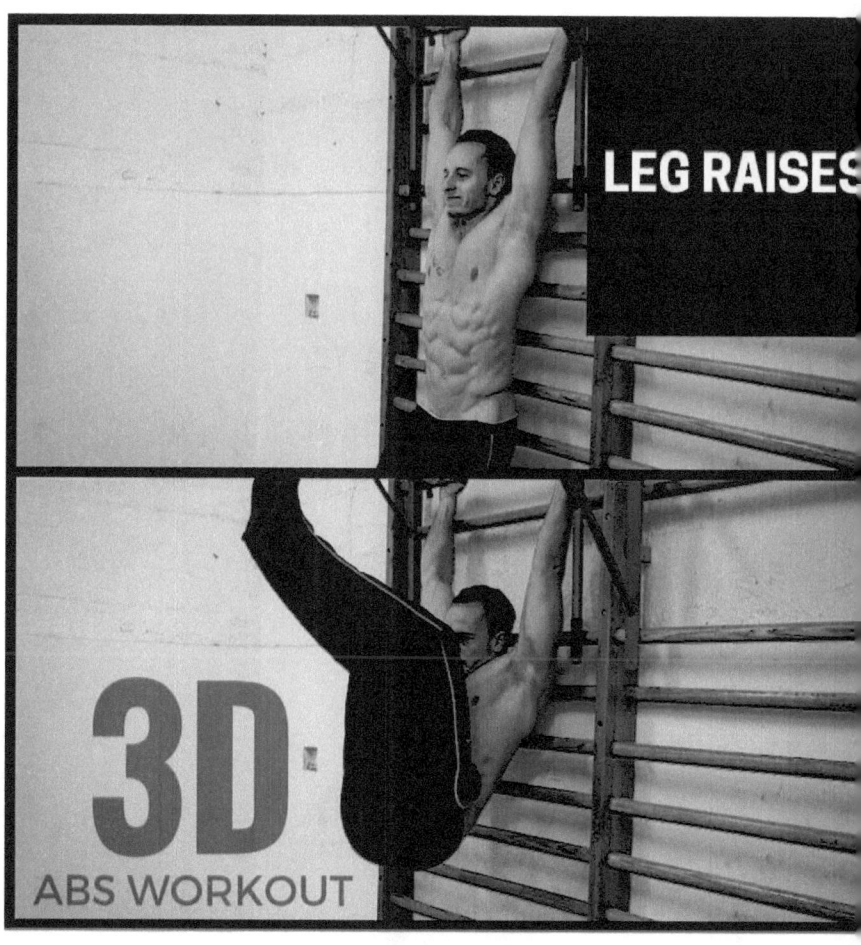

Remember to do full range of motion all the way up. Do not stop in the middle, because you won´t target the majority of your ab muscles. As you get advanced, you shouldn´t go all the way down with your legs anymore. That way you are able to engage your abs all the time.

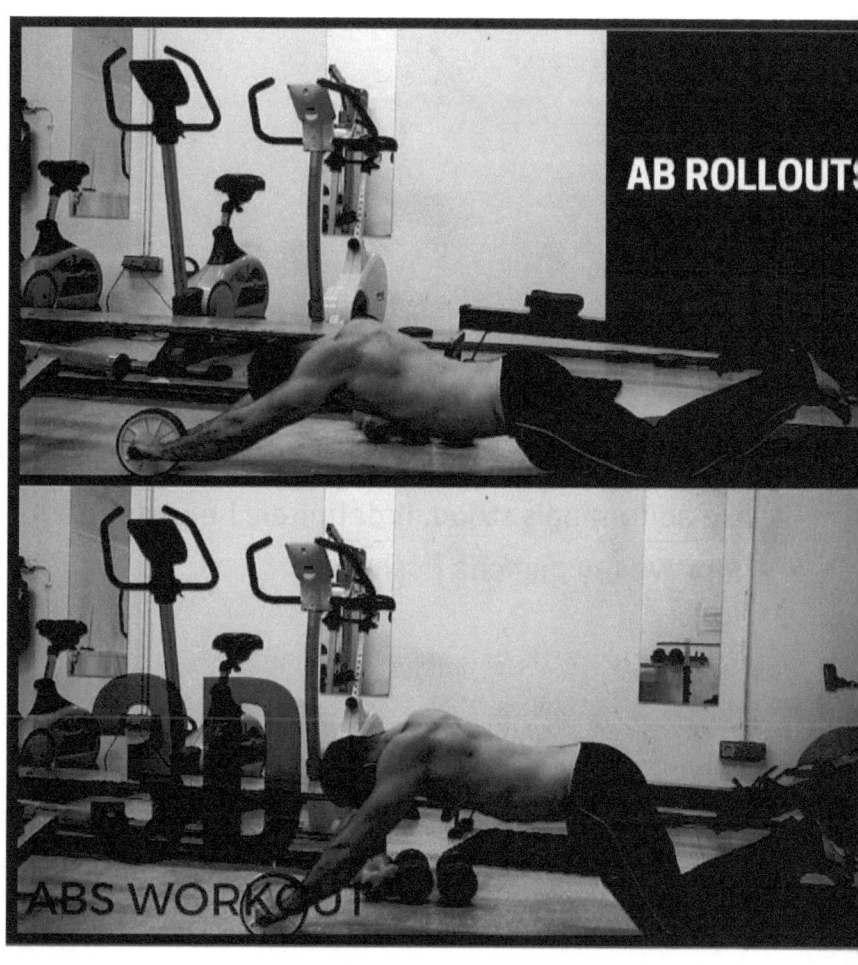

This exercise is great for keeping your core compact and very strong. Don´t go all the way back, but keep the tension on the abs. This exercise is rather advanced so if you are a beginner you don´t have to do this. It is for more advanced guys/girls, who would like to have stone-like abdominals stone. It definitely helped me a lot to improve my planche push-ups.

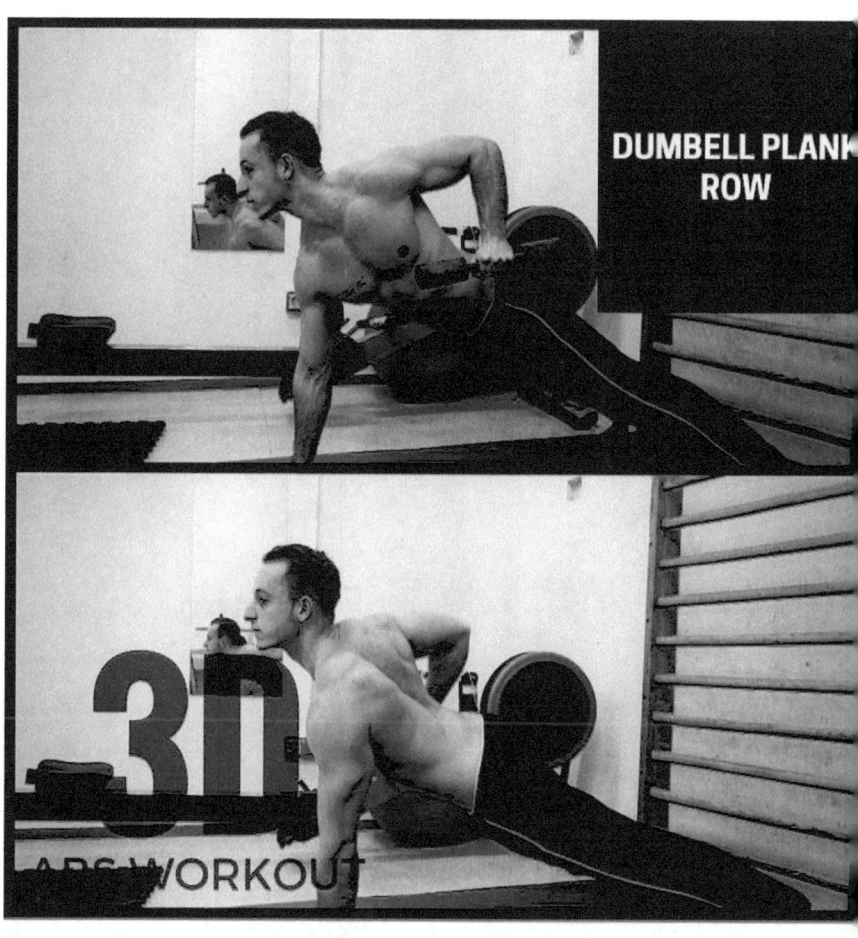

This one helps you increase your punching power, improves core stability and makes your side abs pop out. To make it a little bit harder, try to use heavier dumbbells or simply put your legs onto a higher object like a bench or a box.

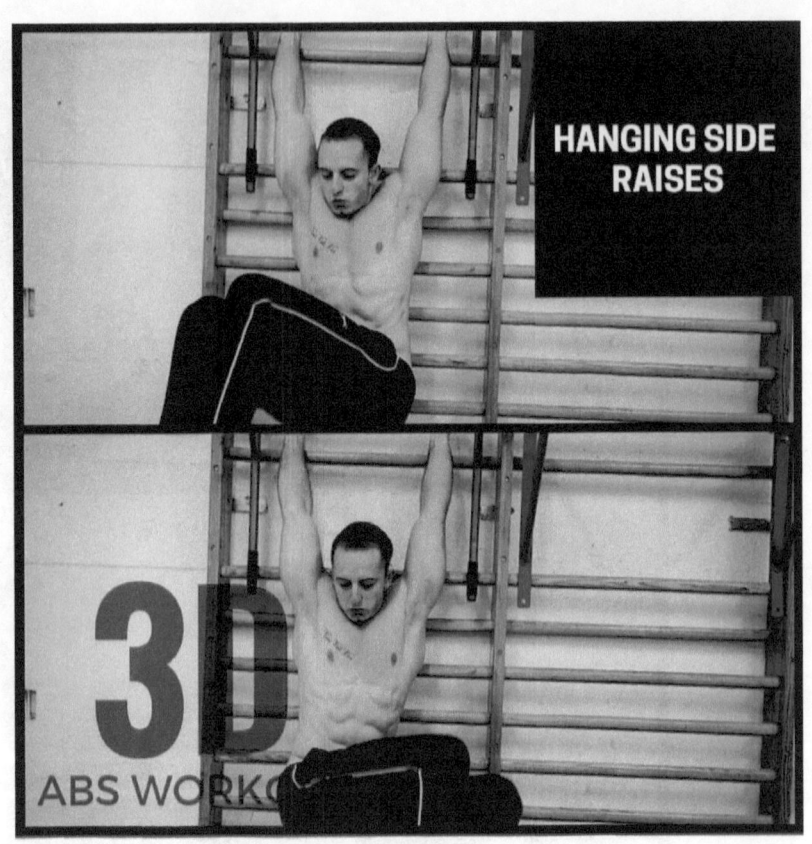

Don´t use momentum here. Simply go from side to side without fully straightening out your legs.

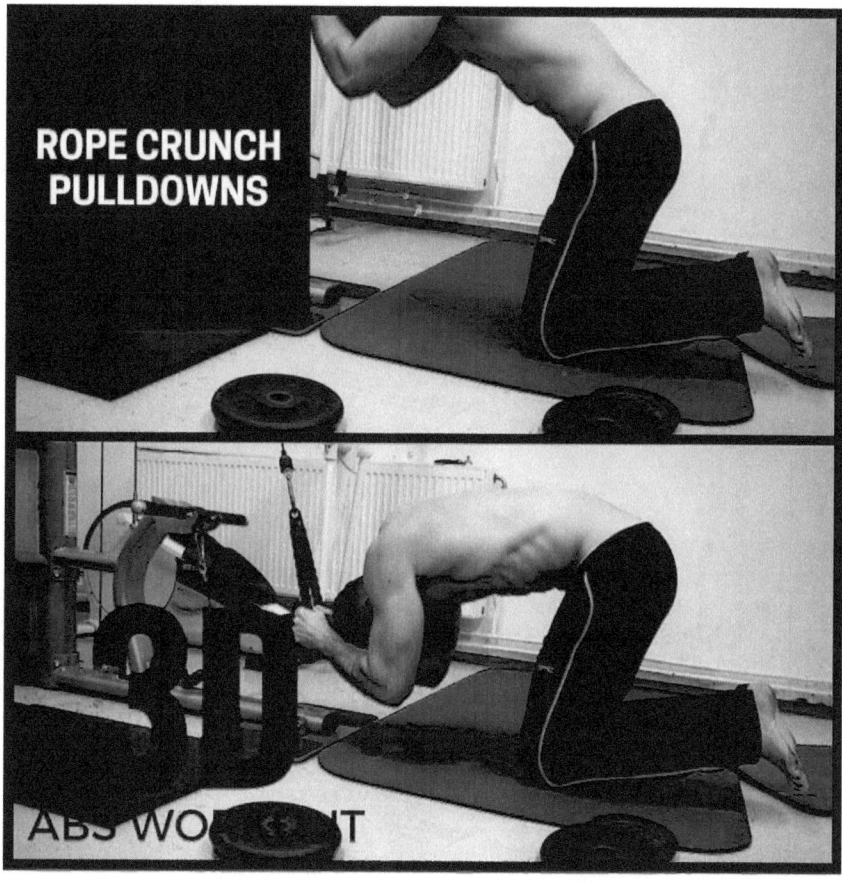

It´s great to go all the way down until you reach your knees with your elbows , however the cable I am using here is too short to enable me such movement.

At the end it doesn´t matter how many of various ab exercises you do but how precise you do them. It is about perfecting the movement which is responsible for the ab contraction. If you keep practicing it while having a great form, you don´t need any other exercises for abs. It is like working out your biceps – you could think of any kind of curl variations for your biceps but at the end it comes down to how well can you perform the curl itself?

Conclusion

Thank you so much for purchasing this book! I am so glad that I could offer you new insights and inform you about intermittent fasting. Even though it is not as mainstream right now as it could be, I think it is going to be really trendy in the following years, just because its great benefits and practicality and because of the whole fitness industry giving people such a hard time preparing their meals and stressing about their diet in general.

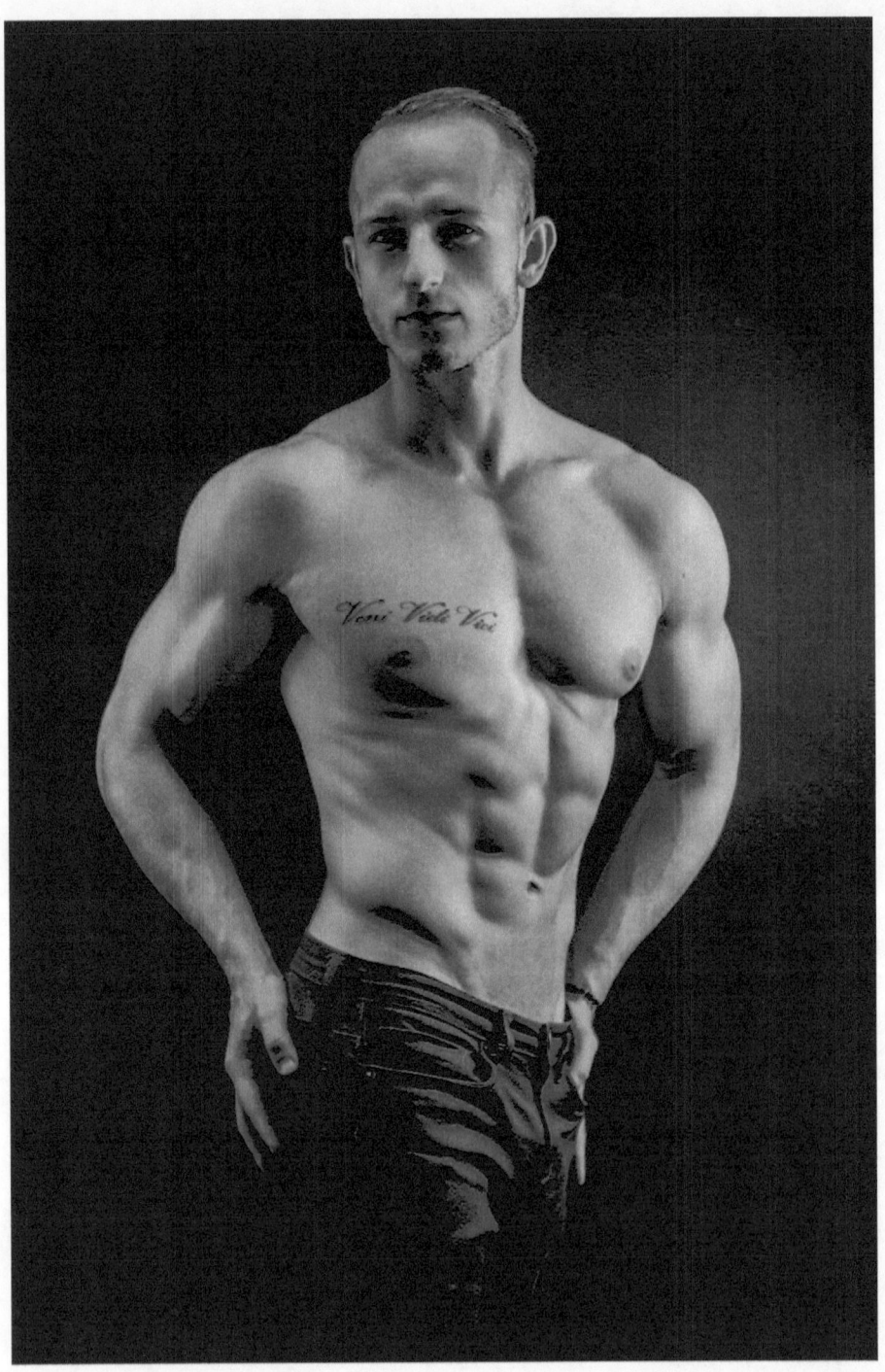

If you enjoyed reading this book, please leave a short review to help this book reach more people and grow its audience!

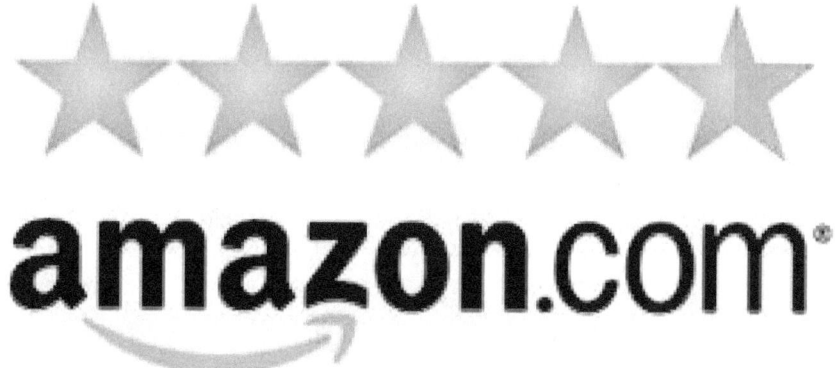

Thank you!